HOW TO GO
ALCOHOL FREE

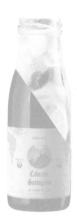

100 TIPS FOR A SOBER LIFE

KATE BEE
THE SOBER SCHOOL

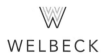

WELBECK

Published in 2019 by Welbeck
An imprint of the Welbeck Publishing Group
20 Mortimer Street
London W1T 3JW

A CIP catalogue for this book is available from the British Library.

ISBN 978-1-78739-346-2

Printed in China

10 9 8 7 6 5 4 3 2 1

CONTENTS

INTRODUCTION

Congratulations for picking up this book! I know that, right now, as you read these words, you might be experiencing many different emotions.

Perhaps you're fed up of feeling hungover and you've been beating yourself up for drinking too much. Maybe you've tried cutting down, but frustratingly, it never seems to work for long.

Perhaps you want to stop, but you're worried about missing out or feeling deprived. Or maybe you're feeling overwhelmed and confused because you don't know where to start. If any of this sounds familiar, don't worry. You are in the right place.

Whether you're trying to quit for good or you're simply curious about exploring an alcohol-free lifestyle, this book is here to make the transition easy for you.

Life is too short to let booze hold you back or make you miserable. After years of drinking too much and feeling bad about it, I decided to go alcohol free in 2013. It's one of the best decisions I've ever made.

I know that if someone like me can do this, you can too. I don't have magic powers or even tons of willpower. I just discovered an approach to alcohol-free living that's really worked for me and my clients.

In this book, I've taken the principles I teach at The Sober School, through my online stop drinking course, Getting Unstuck, and condensed everything down into 100 easy-to-follow tips.

All you need is an open mind and a willingness to try something different. So if you're ready… let's get started. Your alcohol-free adventure is about to begin!

WHERE
TO BEGIN

When it comes to sobriety, a lot of people follow what I call the "wing and a prayer" approach. They stop drinking without a plan and decide to just hope for the best and see what happens. That rarely works out! It's much easier if you have a plan and a goal to work towards. This first chapter will get you focused, fired up and motivated to change – without feeling daunted or overwhelmed.

#1
KNOW THE RISKS

Alcohol is one of the most normalized and widely used drugs on the planet. Because it's sold in pretty bottles and marketed through glamorous, fancy ads, it's easy to overlook just how dangerous booze is for us. So before we go any further, let's be clear on why going alcohol free is such a good idea for your health:

- According to the World Health Organization, alcohol causes one in 20 deaths worldwide.

- In 2018, a large global study published in *The Lancet* concluded there is no "safe" level of alcohol consumption.

- Alcohol is a carcinogen. It causes seven types of cancer, including breast, mouth and bowel cancers.

- Alcohol alters your brain chemistry. Long-term use can lead to a range of mental health issues, such as depression, anxiety, memory loss and even suicide.

#2
DON'T FALL FOR THE OLD WIVES' TALES

At the height of my drinking career, I firmly believed red wine was good for my heart. I clung on to this thought as I poured one glass after another… overlooking the fact that this so-called benefit has been widely debunked.

In 2014, a University of Pennsylvania study concluded that drinking alcohol provides no heart benefit at all, not even when consumed in light amounts. In the UK, the latest government alcohol guidance concluded "there is no justification for drinking for health reasons".

If you search 1950s smoking adverts on the Internet, you'll find all kinds of claims about the benefits of smoking. They seem so silly and outrageous now – why did people ever fall for it? I wonder, in 30 or 40 years' time, whether we'll look back and say the same thing about alcohol.

#3
BRING YOUR VALUES INTO ALIGNMENT

Something I've noticed about the women I coach is that they tend to be health nuts by day and boozers by night. Seeing as you've picked up this book, I'm wondering if you are too.

Perhaps you go to the gym and watch your weight; shun processed foods and avoid refined sugars. Maybe you buy organic, take vitamins, drink green smoothies, guzzle filtered water, count calories and worry about hidden chemicals in your food.

If you care about your health and appearance, it really doesn't make sense to pour a toxic, cancer-causing substance down your neck every night! Don't think of sobriety as "giving something up". Instead, consider it a lifestyle upgrade. By letting go of alcohol, you're simply bringing your values into alignment.

#4
YOU'LL BE IN GOOD COMPANY

Choosing not to use a drug like alcohol doesn't make you weird, it makes you wise – and right on trend! In Britain, the number of teetotallers has risen sharply, with about one in five adults (some 10.4 million people) now abstaining from alcohol. The popularity of months like Dry January and Sober October have normalized the idea of taking time off from drinking, with millions of people taking part.

If you need any more evidence that our drinking patterns are changing, look at the big alcohol brands. Diageo – the world's largest producer of spirits – now owns a stake in the non-alcoholic drinks company Seedlip, and brewer Heineken has launched an alcohol-free version of its flagship beer. These companies aren't producing these drinks on a whim. They're following consumer behaviour and reacting to our changing drinking patterns.

#5
BE HONEST WITH YOURSELF

"Do I really need to stop drinking?" I must have asked myself that question so many times. In the boozy world we live in, working out what's "normal", and what isn't, can be tricky. Here are some signs it's time to take a break:

- You spend a lot of time thinking about drinking – what, where, when, how much?

- You promise to "just have one", but that rarely happens.

- You've created lots of rules in an attempt to control your alcohol intake – e.g. not drinking before a set time, only allowing yourself certain types of drinks.

- You hide the true extent of your drinking from others.

- You feel ashamed of your drinking.

- Your favourite way to drink is by yourself – alone, you can have as much as you like without being judged.

- You're often anxious about whether there's enough alcohol available. Will your supplies last? Should you get more?

- You buy your wine from different shops on rotation because you're worried the store staff will judge you.

- You delay eating so you can drink first without a full stomach dampening your "buzz".

- You rush through things, such as your child's bedtime story, in order to be able to drink.

- You're disappointed – angry, even – if you're unexpectedly asked to be the designated driver and can't drink.

- You're regularly blacking out – there are long periods of time for which you have no memory.

- Mornings often begin with you trying to work out who you called last night and what you said.

- You frequently argue with your partner while drunk, then can't remember why the next day.

- You're exhausted – alcohol is seriously affecting the quality of your sleep.

- You rarely have enough energy for the hobbies you used to love.

- Your physical appearance is changing, your face looks puffier.

- You're scared something bad is going to happen.

- You find yourself reading a book like this.

If you've ticked yes to more than two or three above, you're in the right place. You have absolutely nothing to lose from taking a break from drinking – and so much to gain!

#6
THE MYTH OF ROCK BOTTOM

Perhaps you recognize yourself in the checklist of signs I just outlined, but you're quietly convinced that your drinking isn't yet "bad enough".

Perhaps you've heard about other people's experiences: that time they woke up in hospital, with no memory of how they got there; the moment they got arrested for drink driving, lost a job or ruined a relationship.

Many drinkers believe you need to have a "rock-bottom moment" before you stop drinking – that you have to reach breaking point before you decide to put down the glass.

Let me tell you, that is nonsense! None of us need to be anywhere near rock bottom in order to decide we'll raise our standards and stop hurting ourselves.

#7
DITCH THE LABELS

I'm pretty sure that if you quit smoking, you wouldn't find it necessary to call yourself a "nicotine-oholic". So rest assured, you can quit drinking without having to label yourself an alcoholic.

Sobriety is just about letting go of a habit that's no longer serving you. Personally, I never use the term alcoholic to describe myself. If I have to call myself anything, I go for "alcohol free" because it sounds positive and empowering, which is exactly how it feels!

#8
FLIP YOUR FOCUS

Still not sure if your drinking is "bad enough" for you to need to do something about it? If there's a little part of you that's resisting change, pose a different question. Rather than wondering whether things are bad enough, ask yourself: is my drinking *good enough*?

Given all the downsides to drinking, does alcohol still deserve a place in your life? Are the benefits you're getting from booze enough to outweigh the negatives?

Ultimately, the very fact that you're reading this book is a clue that all is not OK. We both know you're curious about changing things, so don't let any fears you may have stop you from taking action.

#9
COMMIT TO TAKING A BREAK FROM BOOZE

Here's what I'm going to suggest you do next: take a break from booze. Commit to going alcohol free for a defined period of time, so you can test-drive sobriety and find out what it's really all about.

There is absolutely no need to declare that you're quitting "forever". That F-word is sure to trigger so much fear and overwhelm, you might talk yourself out of taking any action at all.

Sobriety is a mindset game. As soon as we start talking about never ever drinking again, our focus shifts to the wrong things and it feels unmanageable.

The beauty of taking a break is that you can treat it like an experiment. You're just seeing what happens when you give alcohol-free living a proper try. Once it's over, you'll review how you feel and decide what to do next. You might go back to drinking, or you might not.

#10
DON'T BE TEMPTED TO MODERATE

When you take your break from booze, the crucial thing is to go all in. Don't be tempted to "just have one" here or there. I'm willing to bet that you've already tried cutting back before and it hasn't worked for long.

Moderation rarely works because it's hard to exercise control over a mind-altering drug that zaps your willpower and destroys your best intentions. We don't expect to be able to "control" our intake of other addictive drugs, so why should we be able to do it with alcohol?

The other problem with moderation is that it reinforces the belief that you cannot enjoy life without alcohol. A big part of successful sobriety is opening your mind to the possibility that life can be lived a little differently.

I know you're reading this book because you've already started to wonder whether alcohol is everything it's cracked up to be – so why not give yourself the opportunity to experience alcohol-free living properly?

#11
WHY TAKING A BREAK WORKS

Taking a proper break from booze means you give yourself the chance to break out of the frustrating pattern a lot of drinkers are stuck in.

When you're only having a few days off each week (e.g. being good Monday to Thursday and then drinking all weekend), you're never experiencing true alcohol-free living. In fact, all you're really doing is making yourself repeat the hardest bit of sobriety (the first few days) over and over again!

Taking a break is also better than taking things "one day at a time". That approach forces you to keep questioning the decision, day in, day out, which is exhausting. With a break, you make that decision only once.

#12
SEE THE BENEFITS

You have so much to look forward to during your break! One of the most visible changes will be the way you look. Alcohol is packed with empty calories, widening your waistline. It also dehydrates your skin, reducing elasticity and increasing redness.

Vogue magazine quoted New York nutritionist Jairo Rodriguez as saying: "Alcohol is actually one of the worst, most aggressive compounds to destroy your skin. I always joke with my patients, 'If you want to get older, go ahead and drink!'"

I strongly recommend you take a selfie before you start your break from alcohol. When women join my stop drinking course, Getting Unstuck, I always get them to do this at the beginning, then they take another one six weeks later. The results are always impressive, but you won't believe it unless you see it, so take that photo!

#13
BECOME RICH!

When you're drinking, you throw money down the drain every day. Booze isn't cheap and even if you're just buying a few bottles here and there, it can quickly add up without you knowing.

Before you start your break from booze, take some time to work out how much alcohol is costing you. Don't forget, you're not just paying for the alcohol itself. You also need to add up the other costs that come with this lifestyle: the hangover food, lost phones, missed days off work, the gym membership you don't use… it really adds up!

Set up a savings account where you transfer the amount you would've spent on booze each week, or put cash into a glass jar as a visual reminder. Don't be afraid to spend this money on treats for yourself – you deserve it!

#14
FEEL HAPPIER

It can seem as if drinking boosts your mood and makes you feel better, but in the long term, the opposite happens. Alcohol is a depressant that's proven to increase stress and anxiety.

Drinking gives you a very brief, artificial high, which is followed by a crushing low afterwards. "Hangxiety" – that morning-after combination of guilt, anxiety and a hangover – is not pleasant. It sets you up for a day of feeling less than your best, which makes you more likely to drink again and repeat the cycle.

Regular drinking lowers the levels of serotonin in your brain, making alcohol and depression a vicious cycle. In sobriety, many of my clients have seen dramatic shifts in their mood, with some being able to come off antidepressants entirely.

#15
SKYROCKET YOUR CONFIDENCE

When you take a complete break from booze for an extended period of time, the chances are you're going to end up sober in some social situations. This is a good thing, because sobriety shouldn't be about living like a loser and never doing fun things!

Being able to socialize without the crutch of alcohol is a really good skill to have, and the chances are you're more confident than you think.

There's something incredibly powerful about going out, having a good time and coming home knowing it was all real – your feelings were 100 per cent genuine and not artificially enhanced in any way.

#16
ENJOY A BETTER WORK-LIFE BALANCE

When you're drinking, your weekends become very short because alcohol is a massive time thief! You lose so much time thinking about drinking, being drunk, feeling hungover and beating yourself up afterwards.

When your weekend isn't lost in a boozy haze, it feels a lot longer. You finally have the time to get stuff done, do the things you enjoy and spend quality time with friends and family. By the time Monday morning rolls around, you feel as if you've had a proper weekend because you have a full, active life outside the workplace.

#17
BE A BETTER PERSON

You know that thing you said you'd help your friend with? The Saturday morning run you've been meaning to do for ages? And that family meal you promised you'd organize? It's really hard to show up for yourself or other people when your days are controlled by a drug that makes you forgetful, sluggish and ultimately not yourself.

Taking a break from booze will make it a lot easier to be the parent, partner and friend you want to be. When you're not hungover, you're more patient. You have more energy. You can run around after the kids. And, most important of all, you get to be fully present for your one and only life.

#18
DECIDE HOW LONG YOUR BREAK WILL BE

So now the big question: how long should your break be for? It's completely up to you, but I recommend doing more than a month if you can.

Studies show you need a minimum of 66 days for a new habit to bed in – and to be honest, one month just isn't really long enough to experience sobriety properly.

Remember, this break from booze isn't about you hiding at home, feeling miserable and avoiding all temptation for the duration. It's about you living your normal life and seeing how it feels to do that, without booze.

Here are some suggested time frames:

- 6 weeks
- 2 months
- 66 days
- 3 months
- 100 days (this has a nice ring to it!)

#19
START BEFORE YOU'RE READY

There is never going to be a "perfect" time to do this. If you look hard enough, there will always be a reason to put your break off: a wedding, a holiday, a birthday, a stressful project at work, your in-laws visiting, etc., etc. There will always be *something* that could get in your way and derail you if you choose to let it.

When you keep putting something off, it starts to feel more and more impossible, and you feel increasingly less ready to do it. Sometimes, you just have to decide that this is the right time and you're going to make it work, no matter what.

You become ready by taking action – not by trying to figure things out from the sidelines. If alcohol is making you miserable, or you suspect it's holding you back in any way at all, the perfect time to quit is always going to be *now*.

#20
DON'T QUESTION THE DECISION

Once you've decided to go for it, make a firm decision, not a flimsy one. Don't say, "I'm going to *try* not to drink during my break." That attitude means that ultimately, booze is still on the table. To-ing and fro-ing over the decision is exhausting and wears you down. It's so much easier to make one firm decision and give it your all – no ifs, buts or maybes.

Apply the teeth-brushing principle. You don't "try" to clean your teeth twice a day, every day. You just do it, right? Even when you've had a bad day, you still find time to do it because you're committed to cleaning your teeth! Treat your break from booze the same way.

Remember, you can always go back to drinking at the end of your break, if you want. But first, you've got to find out what alcohol-free living is really all about. Don't you deserve that opportunity and experience? This break could be life-changing. You have *nothing* to lose.

NAVIGATING EARLY SOBRIETY

In early sobriety, you're bound to experience some cravings for drink, especially around wine o'clock time – or, as some people call it, "the witching hour". It's important to understand that cravings say nothing about you. They're not a sign that you're weak, flawed or destined for failure. They're just a sign that you're changing a habit and you're feeling it. Let's make sure you have all the strategies you need to get off to a flying start!

#21
GET CLEAR ON YOUR "WHY"

When it comes to stopping drinking and staying motivated, one of the best action steps you can take is to figure out your "why". There are going to be some ups and downs, challenges and times when you think "I can't be bothered with this". In those moments when you're close to giving up, knowing your "why" can give you the extra push you need to keep going.

In a journal, make a list of all the reasons motivating you to change. You'll probably find that you start off with obvious things – e.g. "I hate feeling hungover". But as you keep writing, you'll move on to things that are more personal.

"I hate not being able to remember what I said to my partner last night."

"I hate rushing through activities with the kids so I can get back to my drink."

"I hate wondering if people know about my drinking."

Take your time over this list and keep adding to it as you think of more. Make sure you keep this somewhere accessible, so you can return to it during any doubts or wobbles.

#22
HAVE SNACKS AND WATER ON HAND FOR WINE O'CLOCK

It's no coincidence that we feel the strongest urge to drink at the end of the day – a time when we're often hungry, tired and dehydrated. Pouring a glass of wine when you get home from work makes you feel better partly because it's giving you a sugary energy boost just when you're flagging.

The good news is, you can give yourself that same boost through food and water – it's a really simple way to take care of cravings. Carry a bottle of water with you and set a reminder on your phone so you remember to drink it. Keep a healthy snack on hand to help ease any hunger pangs. If you're struggling, some dried fruit or sweets will help ward off cravings until you have your evening meal.

#23
BUILD A SOBER TOOLBOX

A tool is anything you use as a coping mechanism, to change or relieve the way you feel. Until now you've been using alcohol as a tool to help you deal with certain emotions. One of the keys to successful sobriety is to find new, healthier tools that do the same kind of job, but without any of the negative consequences.

Your sober toolbox is what you'll turn to when you need help to change your mood or navigate difficult emotions without drinking.

It's completely up to you what goes in your sober toolbox. Don't worry about being perfect. While it would be great if your sober tools included yoga and meditation, it's also fine to binge-watch Netflix and eat ice cream, if that's what you're in the mood for. The most important thing is that you're not drinking!

Examples of sober tools:
- Taking an exercise class
- A brisk walk outside
- Playing with your pet
- Talking to a friend
- A long bath
- A cup of tea and a good book
- Watching your favourite show

#24
PLAN, PLAN, PLAN

In early sobriety, winging it or "seeing how it goes" rarely works. I know planning doesn't sound very sexy, but when we're boy scouts about this and come prepared, it sets us up for success. For you, planning ahead might mean deciding in advance what you're going to do on Friday evening, if that's a tricky night for you, and making a plan for how you'll handle any cravings.

It might mean working out what your soft drink options are in the pub, deciding what you'll say to friends, or whether you should go in the first place. Planning ahead gives you the opportunity to troubleshoot any potential problems and give yourself the best chance of success.

#25
TACKLE ONE THING AT A TIME

When you're excited about turning over a new leaf, it's easy to get carried away. But now isn't the time to put yourself on a punishing new diet or start an extreme fitness regime. We all have a finite supply of time, energy and willpower. Right now, alcohol-free living needs 100 per cent of your attention.

Take it easy on yourself and focus on mastering this one thing. Alcohol is packed with empty calories, so by losing the booze, you're already making one diet-savvy move. And when you're not hungover, the chances are you'll naturally be a bit more active anyway. There's no need to force yourself to do anything else just yet. All in good time!

#26
DO YOUR SOBER HOMEWORK

A great way to stay focused and keep your head in the game is to bookend your day with a sobriety-related activity or routine. So, first thing in the morning, you could listen to a podcast about sobriety as you get ready for the day or commute to work. In the evening you could keep a journal, or read some sober blogs or a memoir about alcohol-free living before you go to bed. This practice will help you start and close each day in the right mindset.

#27
PLAY THE MOVIE TO THE END

When a craving strikes, it's all too easy to get caught up in the moment. The next time you feel an urge to drink, imagine your drinking as a story. You're at the start of the movie right now and you get to decide the storyline. If you choose to drink, how is the movie going to end? Set a timer on your phone for two minutes and force yourself to think things through, hour by hour.

This exercise requires brutal honesty in order to work properly. You have to force yourself to imagine what will *really* happen if you have "just one" drink. The chances are that if you have one glass of wine, you'll go on to have two, three or four more. I don't think you'd be reading this if you were the kind of person who just has one! If you drink, how will you feel when you wake up, physically and mentally? You will be kicking yourself. It's never worth it.

#28
FLIP THE STORYLINE

Now switch things around and think about what will happen if you *don't* drink. Cravings will and do pass – and the good news is, we're talking about minutes rather than hours. If you can just sit this out for a short while, you will soon feel better. Now's the time to raid your sober toolbox, distract yourself and wait for the urge to pass.

Picture how nice it will be to go to bed with a clear head instead of feeling blurry and drunk. You'll have a great night's sleep before waking up in the morning, proud, refreshed and ready to tackle the day. That's the kind of movie we all want to have, right?

#29
PICTURE YOUR CRAVINGS AS A MONSTER

Visualize yourself feeding this monster whenever you drink and starving it when you don't – because this really is what you're doing! Every time you drink, you're feeding that mental and emotional craving for alcohol. You're putting alcohol back into your body, back into your system, and that just makes things harder physically.

Know that every time you make it through a craving and do not give in, you're destroying a little bit more of this monster. Visualize it suffocating, starving and getting physically smaller.

It's reassuring to know that this *will* get easier with time. Right now you're killing the monster, and things won't be this hard forever.

#30
LISTEN TO YOUR CRAVINGS

Cravings nearly always have something to tell us – they're a sign that something is off. Our body is simply trying to get us to pay attention and address a problem. So rather than interpreting that craving as a cue to drink, tune back into your body and work out what it is you really need.

Perhaps you're hungry or thirsty. Maybe you're tired, stressed out or overwhelmed. Could you be bored, lonely or feeling a bit sad? Get curious about what the craving is telling you and then think about what sober tools you could use to help yourself feel better. Perhaps you need to talk to a friend, jump in the bath for some "me time" or get an early night. When you listen and take action to remedy the problem, you'll soon feel better.

#31
MIX THINGS UP

If you're struggling to identify what's wrong, or perhaps you just feel a bit "off", focus on changing things up instead – it can help snap you out of a downward spiral. Get outside and go for a walk, so you change your surroundings. Physical exercise and time in nature is always great.

If you can't switch your surroundings, change your mood. A warm bath will help you relax and a cold shower will shift your focus. Listening to music or watching a film will distract you, and calling a friend will help you change the conversation you're having in your head.

#32
DON'T FORGET SELF-CARE

For many people – especially women – the only time they let themselves stop, relax and do nothing is when they're drinking. We live in a world where wine is often promoted as "self-care" – it's the start of "me time" and a signal to relax and switch off.

In sobriety, don't assume that just because you're not drinking, you've lost that permission to do nothing and relax. Sobriety doesn't mean always being "on" – no one can survive like that for long. Recovery isn't punishment (you've done enough of that already). We all need rest and relaxation, and you absolutely deserve to chill out like you used to!

Self-care isn't about self-improvement, nor is it just manicures and facials. It's really about looking after yourself at a deep level. If you found the time to drink, you can definitely find time to do something nice for yourself like reading a book, taking a bath or watching a bit of TV. It doesn't need to be complicated, it just needs to make you feel good.

#33
FIND A TRIBE

We humans are social creatures – we're wired for connection. While you can stop drinking on your own, with just this book for company, it can be rather lonely at times. It is so much easier when you have people to talk to about this, to cheer you on and help you troubleshoot the tricky times.

At The Sober School, my stop drinking course is a group coaching programme for a reason: I know how powerful it is to take this journey with other people. Being part of a motivated, inspiring community can really help things click into place. You are not the only person in the world to struggle with alcohol and it's important you know that.

So where can you find support? Here are some ideas:

- Look around you. Perhaps you already have people in your life who don't drink or who would wholeheartedly support you. Be brave – reach out for support and take a risk.

- Start a blog. You can set up a free and anonymous blog on WordPress. Start following other bloggers and, chances are, they'll follow you back. Writing can be a great way to make sense of your thoughts.

- Find a Facebook group. There are lots of alcohol-related support groups on Facebook, which you can request to join.

- Try an AA (Alcoholics Anonymous) meeting. Personally, AA was never my cup of tea, but I do think it's a great way to meet people in your area who are on a similar journey.

- Come and join The Sober School! I run my stop drinking course every few months and I'd love to have you in my tribe. If you go to thesoberschool.com, you can sign up to the waiting list and find out more.

#34
MAKE SURE YOU HAVE SOMETHING LOVELY TO DRINK

I feel very strongly that sobriety should not be about making do with rubbish drinks! Being alcohol free does not mean you have to put up with boring tap water or flat Diet Coke. You're an adult – you deserve grown-up, delicious drinks just like everyone else.

The good news is, there has never been a better range of options for non-drinkers. From alcohol-free spirits, beers and wines to glamorous mocktails, there's so much to choose from. A quick search for mocktail recipes will bring up more ideas than you know what to do with!

My all-time favourite drink is fresh grapefruit juice mixed with slimline tonic water. I also love elderflower cordial with sparkling water, and tonic water with Seedlip (an alcohol-free spirit). I make sure I serve everything in a nice, grown-up wine glass – it has to look good as well as taste good!

#35

ALCOHOL-FREE WINES AND BEERS ARE FINE

A lot of people wonder whether it's "OK" to consume alcohol-free versions of their favourite drinks. In the sober community, these drinks are controversial and some people have strong views on whether they're a good idea. Personally, I think they're absolutely fine. If they work for you, go for it!

I have many clients who find these drinks to be a total lifesaver. They enjoy the taste and it stops them feeling as if they're missing out. However, I also know other people who find these drinks to be a bit too close to the real deal and that makes them uncomfortable.

Don't let anyone else tell you what's wrong or right on this. If you're curious about them, try one and see how it feels. You'll probably have a gut feeling about whether they're your thing or not.

#36
GET A NATURAL BUZZ

When you get into the habit of drinking too much, it's easy to forget that there are natural highs out there. If you're craving a healthy high to replace the buzz you got from alcohol, here are some ideas:

- Exercise. It releases endorphins, which are sometimes referred to as "natural morphine" because they spark a positive, euphoric feeling.

- Listen to great music. When we listen to music we love, our brain releases dopamine, a feel-good chemical.

- Get outside more. Exposure to green spaces has been proven to make us happier.

- Laugh more. It relieves tension, helps us bond with others and has a relaxing effect on the whole body for up to 45 minutes afterwards.

#37
MOTHER YOURSELF

Early sobriety can be very challenging, as you relearn how to deal with your emotions and navigate the ups and downs of everyday life, sober. The chances are that it will feel like a roller coaster at times, and the best way to survive this period is to mother yourself.

Look after your new, sober self in the same way that you might take care of a cranky and overwhelmed toddler. So, get plenty of early nights and remember that everything always feels better in the morning. Eat good-quality food. Drink lots of water. Set boundaries and know when to say no. And most of all be kind, patient and understanding with yourself. You're doing something great here!

#38
TREAT YOURSELF!

If alcohol has always been your main luxury or reward, I suspect you've probably fallen out of the habit of looking after yourself in other ways. Now's the time to scoop up the money you're saving on booze and start investing in yourself.

Remember: sobriety isn't about living a life of deprivation. It's about creating an amazing, feel-good life; one that's so great, you don't need to numb your way through it. It's amazing what you can treat yourself to, even on a budget.

Here are some of my favourite sober treats:

- Fresh flowers
- Fancy moisturizers
- A monthly subscription to a magazine, beauty box or cake delivery service
- A cup of tea and a good book
- Good-quality hot chocolate
- A cheeky midweek trip to the cinema
- New pyjamas
- Getting my hair blow-dried
- A fancy alcohol-free cocktail

#39
DON'T WORRY ABOUT DRINKING DREAMS

It's alarming to wake up in a cold sweat, convinced you've been drinking all night. Some people have drinking dreams so vivid and real they feel very upset by them. Drinking dreams are very common in early sobriety, but don't worry – they're not a sign you are about to slip up.

When something is important to us, we think about it a lot. And when something's on our mind, it often shows up in our dreams too. While these drinking dreams are unpleasant, they do serve quite a useful function; they are a reminder of how you'd feel if you really did drink.

#40
KNOW THAT THE ROAD AHEAD IS EASIER

Do you remember learning to drive? It seemed impossible at first, right? There were so many things to think about: moving into the right gear, keeping your eyes on the road and remembering to mirror, signal, manoeuvre. It felt clunky, exhausting and stressful at times.

Early sobriety is a bit like learning to drive. Right now, it's going to require a fair bit of brain power and energy. You're bound to be thinking about sobriety a lot and it probably doesn't feel very natural, yet. I promise it soon will do. Keep going – this is all going to be so worth it!

SOCIALIZING AND DEALING WITH OTHER PEOPLE

If you announced you were quitting smoking, no one would bat an eyelid – in fact, they'd probably congratulate you! Yet when it comes to alcohol, people don't always respond with quite the same enthusiasm. I think alcohol might be the only drug on the planet that you have to justify *not* taking! This chapter is all about how to deal with other people, so you can socialize sober while keeping your sanity, and still have a great night out.

#41
KEEP THINGS IN PERSPECTIVE

Choosing not to pour a toxic, cancer-causing drug down your neck shouldn't be a big deal. It is fundamentally a very reasonable thing to do! In a world where we're used to people quitting smoking, cutting out gluten and going vegan, going alcohol free should be perfectly normal. I find it very frustrating that some people still think it's OK to pressure others into drinking – we'd never do that with other drugs, right?

When you really think about it, there's nothing "normal" about drinking. Alcohol is a poison that slows down your brain function. Side effects include nausea, vomiting, lethargy, headaches, tremors, heart palpitations and seizures. The fact that we choose to do this to ourselves – and we've made it culturally acceptable and cool to do so – is entirely *abnormal*. It should be sobriety that's considered "normal"!

#42
DON'T ASK FOR OTHER PEOPLE'S OPINIONS ON YOUR DRINKING

The only person who *really* knows how much you're drinking is you. And the only person who truly understands how alcohol makes you feel, is you! It's almost impossible for friends and family to offer an informed, neutral opinion, so don't waste your time asking for it.

Think of it this way: if those around you also drink, then they're much more likely to think that your alcohol intake is fine. There's a lot of bad information about booze out there, and different people have different ideas about what's OK. It's not helpful to expose yourself to that misinformation.

Instead of asking for their opinion, tell your friends and family about your decision once you've made it. Then the only thing you need to ask for is their love and support.

#43
TREAT OTHER PEOPLE'S REACTIONS WITH CAUTION

The way other people respond to your sobriety can be very revealing. It says everything about them – and their relationship with alcohol – and very little about you. When people respond in a negative or judgemental way, you can pretty much guarantee they're feeling defensive or self-conscious about their own drinking.

All you can do in these situations is be patient and compassionate. If you've kept the true extent of your drinking hidden, some people may just be surprised and respond in a clumsy way without thinking.

True friends will adjust to your sobriety fairly quickly – after all, they should like you because of who you are, not what's in your glass! If someone keeps giving you a hard time for not drinking, perhaps they aren't the right person to have in your life anyway.

#44
GET YOUR RESPONSES READY

You don't owe anyone an explanation for why you're not drinking. You certainly don't need to share your life story or drinking history with them. However, you might like to prepare some simple responses (or excuses!) in case people ask you directly. Here are some ideas:

- I don't feel like drinking today

- I'm doing a no-alcohol challenge with friends

- I've been getting too many hangovers / headaches, so I'm taking a break

- Drinking really interferes with my sleep

- I'm driving

- I'm on a diet / doing a detox

- I'm training for a race

- I'm not feeling very well

Whatever response you choose, say it with confidence. Make it clear the decision has already been made and be really positive about it – don't apologize! You don't owe anyone an apology. Make it clear that you're happy not to be drinking. You could even tell people that you're surprised by how good you feel – that way it's harder for them to pester you into having "just one".

#45
IF YOU LIVE WITH SOMEONE WHO DRINKS

Make sure your partner knows what's going on. Even if they don't want to join you for a break from booze, tell them about your plan. Not only does that give you some real-life accountability, but it reduces the chance of them offering you booze by accident. You don't want a glass of wine to be thrust in your hand the minute you get home.

Be brave and outline some boundaries. We're not always very good at asking for things we need, but it is entirely reasonable for you to ask your partner to drink elsewhere, if that's what you need right now. I'm sure that if your partner was trying to lose weight or quit smoking you would be supportive and wouldn't leave temptation lying around.

If your partner isn't being very supportive, find other people to talk to. This is another reason to make sure you're part of a sober tribe and have a supportive community around you. (See Tip 33.)

Most important of all, remember that you are your own person. I'm sure you and your partner already have different tastes, different hobbies and different opinions on many other things. This is no different. You get to choose whether or not you let your partner's drinking hold you back.

#46
TAKE ON THOSE CHALLENGES

During your break from booze, the chances are that you will have to navigate a few social events, whether it's drinks in the pub, a party or meal with friends. Now, perhaps you'll be surprised to hear me say this, but I strongly recommend you continue with your regular social life.

If you empty your calendar and resign yourself to staying at home and avoiding all social contact until your break is over, you will feel deprived. You also won't challenge yourself or learn just how much you're capable of doing without booze.

Successful sobriety is about living your normal life, just without the booze. *That* is how you experience sobriety properly. So lean into the challenges – it's how you make big progress.

#47
DECIDE YOU'RE NOT GOING TO DRINK

I know this sounds kind of obvious, but it's important. The chances are that during your break from booze, there will be a little voice in your head wondering whether a particular night out or social event could be an exception... perhaps you could just have one or two and it wouldn't count?

That voice in your head might convince you to just "wait and see" how you feel when you get there. Don't do that! When you keep the possibility of drinking on the table, you're forcing yourself to do a lot of decision-making on the fly, when you're surrounded by drinkers and booze. This is why a "maybe" nearly always ends up being a yes.

Make the decision that you're not drinking before you go out. Revisit the list you made of all the reasons why you're taking this break. Remind yourself how important this is. Make your sobriety a non-negotiable and do not let the wine witch win!

#48

BE PREPARED TO LEARN SOMETHING NEW ABOUT YOURSELF

If you haven't been to a party sober since you were a teenager, chances are that quite a lot has changed since then! Perhaps you remember your younger self feeling awkward or shy when socializing, and so you've relied on alcohol to ease the wheels of conversation ever since. But what if that old story you have about yourself is just that – an old, outdated story?

I bet your confidence has grown a lot since your teenage years and you're better at making conversation and meeting new people. Be prepared to surprise yourself – you probably don't need alcohol as much as you thought. It's incredibly empowering to realize that you can socialize sober and have a good time, regardless of what's in your glass.

#49
REMEMBER, YOU SOCIALIZE SOBER ALL THE TIME...

You might feel worried at the thought of going out and not drinking, but have you actually stopped to consider how often you socialize sober, without even realizing it? I bet it's more than you think!

Most of us think nothing of catching up with friends over coffee. We banter with our workmates during the day and go out for lunch, sober. We strike up conversation with strangers at business events or chat to people in our yoga class.

All day long, we manage to socialize with other humans, stone-cold sober – and that means we can do exactly the same thing in the evening too.

#50
LEARN FROM
THE KIDS

If you need some inspiration, take a look at the way children behave at parties. They often arrive feeling shy, but within a few minutes they overcome their nerves. Soon they're singing, dancing and making friends. They use genuine courage to break through their fears and soon they're on a natural high, having fun and feeling happy.

We'd be horrified if our children needed to drink in order to have fun. So at what point did we decide that it was different for us adults? Why do we believe that we need to take a mind-altering drug in order to let our hair down and spend time with friends we like? It doesn't make sense!

#51
LEARN TO TRANSLATE

People can often seem more obsessed with alcohol than they really are, because it's a big part of how we communicate. You might hear things like:

"We must go for drinks!"
"I hope to see you again in the bar later."
"I'll bring a bottle of wine round and we can catch up."

Don't let the alcohol references alienate you – instead, learn to listen to what's really being said. Most of the time what people are trying to say is:

"I'd like to spend some time with you."
"It was great meeting you – I'd like to get to know you better."
"It's been ages since I've seen you. Let's spend some quality time together."

We can all be shy sometimes, so instead of saying what we really mean, it can feel easier to make it sound as if all we want is a drink! In reality, what we're truly craving is human connection. Going for a drink is just a vehicle to facilitate that.

#52
KNOW WHAT AN EVENT IS REALLY ALL ABOUT

In this crazy, boozy world of ours, it's easy to build something up in our minds as being entirely about alcohol. When you're not drinking, that kind of thinking leaves you feeling left out. Yet the reality is that parties are about humans coming together for a reason. No event is ever *just* about booze.

If you're feeling worried or fearful, make a mental list of everything the event is really about. For example:

"This party is about old friends getting together."
"This meal is about getting to know my work colleagues better."
"This networking event is about meeting new people."
"This date night is about spending quality time with my partner."

#53
PRACTISE VISUALIZATION

Olympic athletes have been using visualization techniques for decades – it's the equivalent of a mental warm-up! By "brain rehearsing" a positive experience and picturing success, they can increase their chance of achieving a successful outcome in real life. You can do exactly the same thing.

Close your eyes and take some deep breaths in and out. Picture yourself feeling happy and confident. What are you wearing? What can you see? What will you be doing? Visualize yourself making conversation easily, mingling with other people and confidently ordering an alcohol-free drink.

Visualization also gives you the chance to anticipate any challenges. I remember, early in my sobriety, going to a work event where I knew there was going to be free prosecco. Because I'd anticipated this, I wasn't thrown off track by having a glass thrust toward me. Instead I was able to confidently say, "What alcohol-free options do you have?" and they got me something else very quickly.

#54
PLAN YOUR DRINKS IN ADVANCE

Make life easy for yourself by thinking about what you'll drink before you go out. If you're trying to be discreet about your sobriety, tonic water with a slice of lemon is always a good option. If you're going to a bar, check them out online first – do they have an alcohol-free drinks menu? It can be helpful to know what they serve in advance, because you can't always see what's available when you're jostling to get served at a busy bar.

If you're going to a party, let the host know you're not drinking before you arrive. There's nothing more awkward than having to clutch a glass of water all night because no one thought about providing any alcohol-free options. That kind of situation makes everyone feel bad – you feel self-conscious and the host feels as if they're not doing a good job. Having the drinks conversation in advance means that (a) expectations are already set and (b) you actually get a nice drink! You can always offer to bring along something you know you like.

#55
CREATE A MINI TOOLBOX

In Tip 23 I suggested you build a sober toolbox to help you deal with the ups and downs of life without alcohol. It's really handy to have a mini version of this ready to use when you're out and about, in case you're struggling. Whether you're finding a party tough going, or a bad day at work is making you crave wine, it helps to have something close by to keep you on track.

Your mini toolbox could be a little make-up bag where you keep a copy of your list of reasons why you're taking a break from booze. Essential oils, sweets, teabags and inspiring mantras or quotes can be very soothing. Stick some headphones in there too, so you can listen to an audiobook or some inspiring music on your phone.

#56
REMEMBER, YOU DON'T *HAVE* TO GO

The fact that you've made it this far into the book shows that you're pretty committed to changing your drinking – and I hope I've persuaded you that taking a proper break from booze is the right thing to do. It could be absolutely life-changing.

When you are 100% committed to making this break happen, your sobriety is going to be your number-one priority. Putting your sobriety first sometimes means saying no to things. If you're not in the right frame of mind, or you're worried you'll end up drinking – don't go. Stay at home.

How you feel is going to change all the time. I remember going to a really boozy party early in my sobriety and it was absolutely fine – I was in a great mood that day and feeling confident. But a few days later, I skipped another event because I wasn't feeling quite so good.

Not turning up is no big deal – other people do it all the time. It doesn't make you a loser, it's just the right thing to do sometimes. You're doing life-changing work here. It's much smarter (and braver) to know yourself and put your own needs first.

#57
PREPARE AN ESCAPE PLAN

It's fine to leave an event early if you're finding things hard or simply not enjoying yourself. Chances are, most people won't notice and even if they do, who cares? You came and now you're going. Nothing is more important than your sobriety and taking this break from booze.

Make sure you have a way of getting home easily. Offering to drive is a great idea because then you're in control. Even if you're the host of an event and can't leave, you can still escape for breaks when you need them. Go to another room, head out for a short walk or pretend to make a phone call. Do what you need to do and don't feel bad about it!

#58
KEEP AN OPEN MIND

Alcohol can hide a lot of flaws. Once you're not drinking, you may find there are certain places, people or events that you don't love *quite* as much as you thought you did. This can be unsettling, I know, but please don't worry. It's actually a useful discovery!

Here's the thing: if you need a mind-altering substance in order to enjoy a situation, or tolerate certain people, you're not really having a good time, are you? You're not genuinely enjoying it. Personally, I'd much rather know when a situation is boring me. Life's too short to be spending time with people we don't really like or doing things we find dull.

#59
PLAN ALTERNATIVES

In his book *Chasing the Scream*, Johann Hari states that, "The opposite of addiction is connection." I love this perspective. We're wired for connection – when we feel isolated and alone, it can make us miserable.

If you've decided to play it safe and skip a boozy party, make sure you organize something else to do instead. Arrange to meet friends for lunch, catch up over coffee, go for a walk, plan a shopping trip or a cinema date. Take control. Don't hide away, feeling isolated or left out. You don't need to be.

#60
CELEBRATE!

No matter what happens, make sure you reward yourself. Whether you've navigated a tricky event or made the decision not to go, you deserve a treat. A favourite dessert, a good book and fresh sheets on your bed are lovely things to come home to. Take the time to acknowledge and praise yourself for the effort you're putting into this break from booze. You're stepping out of your comfort zone and working on something really important here. Well done!

MINDSET
MATTERS

Alcohol is unlike any other drug because it's so glamorized, romanticized and normalized. The message we often hear from adverts, social media and those around us is that this drug is essential to living a full and happy life. This couldn't be further from the truth! This chapter is all about keeping your mindset in the right place, so can you feel good about taking a break from this toxic, cancer-causing poison.

#61
EDUCATE YOURSELF ABOUT ALCOHOL

When it comes to other aspects of our health, most of us are incredibly knowledgeable. We spend a fortune on superfoods, guzzle filtered water, wear fitness trackers, buy organic and worry about the chemicals in our sunscreen. And yet when it comes to booze, we know shockingly little about it.

Did you realize that alcohol – or ethanol, to give it its proper name – goes into the fuel we use in our cars? Most drinkers have no idea what they're really pouring down their throats. Ethanol is a key ingredient in engine fuel, antiseptics, paints, perfume and deodorants. So it has its uses, for sure ... but why on earth are we pumping our bodies full of it? Don't we deserve *better* than what goes into floor cleaner?

#62
DON'T ROMANTICIZE ROTTING FRUIT JUICE

An entire industry has been built around portraying wine as something elegant and sophisticated, with "fruity notes" and "buttery textures". Don't fall for this clever marketing trap! Most people aren't really drinking for the taste – they're drinking to get drunk.

Have you ever noticed that there are no ingredients listed on the back of wine bottles? Zero. This gives the impression that all wine contains are some innocent, mashed-up grapes, but this couldn't be further from the truth. Modern-day wine production has less to do with sunlit chateaux and more to do with laboratories and scientists in white coats. Wine is packed full of manufactured chemicals, even the organic stuff.

#63
CREATE A POWERFUL ANCHOR

It can be really helpful to have a visual image that snaps you back to reality, should you start to get caught up in a craving. Decide what the picture will be now, so you have it tucked away at the back of your mind. Perhaps you have a particular memory of you doing something you regret. Or maybe there's a picture of you drinking that makes you cringe with embarrassment whenever you see it. Get clear on the details of this image and how you felt in that particular moment. Drinking can seem so glamorous at times, but it's anchors like this that remind us of the true reality.

#64
LEAN INTO YOUR FEAR

When we push ourselves to try new things, like sobriety, it's inevitable that fear will crop up at some point. That's OK. In fact, it's really normal. The important thing to know is that fear isn't a sign you're doing the wrong thing or that you should just give up. The things we're most scared of doing tend to be the things we need to do the most.

As the author Steven Pressfield wrote in *The War of Art*, "The more scared we are of a work or calling, the more sure we can be that we have to do it." Rather than letting yourself be paralyzed by fear, use it as a sign that something precious is at stake; it means you're working on something that really matters. You are doing the right thing!

#65
REFRAME DISCOMFORT

Taking a break from booze is going to push you outside your comfort zone. I know there will be times when it all feels too much, and giving up seems like the easier, safer option. But here's what I want you to remember: drinking only feels "easier" because it's familiar to you. That's all. When you really think about it, drinking isn't actually a very easy thing to do – hangovers, shame and regrets are tough, horrible things to deal with!

Sobriety *is* going to create some discomfort for you, as you try something different and step outside your comfort zone. However, if you stay stuck and carry on drinking, you're also going to experience a lot of discomfort.

So, if you're going to be uncomfortable no matter what you do, why not choose sobriety? You already know what happens when you drink. But you don't yet know what happens when you stick with sobriety. Trust me, it's going to get easier and it will be *so* worth it.

#66
YOUR RELATIONSHIP WITH ALCOHOL SAYS NOTHING ABOUT YOU

Guess what? It's *normal* to become addicted to an addictive substance. It's hard to control a mind-altering drug that zaps your willpower and destroys your best intentions. As a sobriety coach, I've worked with chief executives, high-flying lawyers and busy mums who juggle 101 things every day. There is absolutely no correlation between your strength of character and your relationship with alcohol.

So please, don't for a second think that heavy drinkers are "weak". Personally, I think you have to be quite a tough person to be able to drink and cope with the side effects. Dealing with a killer hangover, while juggling your regular life and trying to pretend everything's hunky-dory, is really hard. Deciding that you're going to change and do something different? That also requires courage.

#67
ALCOHOL ISN'T VERY SMART

Pause for a moment and consider all the different things we're told alcohol can do for us. On some days, it's supposed to give us a bit of a pick-me-up. It makes us lively and more fun to be around. And yet on other days, the exact same liquid drug supposedly has the opposite effect and makes us calm and relaxed. And on other days, it does something different again: it makes us brave, confident and more courageous.

How can alcohol do that? How can it create one effect on one day, and then do the exact opposite on another? Alcohol wasn't invented by top scientists in a high-tech, state-of-the-art lab, so it can't possibly figure out how you're feeling and then respond accordingly!

Alcohol is just a crude, toxic poison that's been around for centuries. The only thing that changes is what we believe alcohol is going to do for us. Our minds are incredibly powerful.

#68
CHALLENGE YOUR BELIEFS ABOUT BOOZE

Willpower alone will only get you so far. To really enjoy sobriety, and feel good about alcohol-free living, you will need to change your thinking about booze. This is the secret to making sobriety feel like a positive, empowering choice.

During my stop drinking course, Getting Unstuck, I help students break down every single "benefit" to drinking that they can put forward. We analyze each one in detail and look at whether they're really true. For example, if you're convinced that alcohol makes you happy and helps you have fun, how do you explain the times when you've drunk lots and not felt good? Or perhaps you felt upset or got into an argument? If alcohol really is some kind of magic joy juice, shouldn't it work every time?

Start analyzing your thoughts and assumptions. What are you telling yourself about alcohol's powers, day in, day out? On a piece of paper, list all the reasons why you've been drinking. Then go through your list point by point and write down evidence that shows this benefit either isn't true, or isn't guaranteed.

#69
DON'T FALL FOR THE STRESS MYTH

One of the most common misconceptions about alcohol is that it helps you cope with stress. We often hear people talking about "relaxing" with a drink at the end of a tough day. However, if alcohol really did fix stress, surely all drinkers would be carefree, easy-going types? And surely they would need less alcohol over time, not more?

Opening a bottle at wine o'clock will not help you cope or deal with stress. Stress happens for a variety of different reasons, and alcohol is just, well, ethanol. It can't possibly make your boss nicer, your children behave better, or your partner more considerate. In short, it can't fix things.

All alcohol can do is distract us and numb us, for a very short time. And that makes it easier to ignore whatever's happening right in front of us. But that's it. Alcohol doesn't solve anything. When we sober up, the exact same problems will still be there – only now you have a hangover to contend with on top of everything else.

#70
ALCOHOL WILL MAKE STRESS WORSE

Consider your own experience here. The problems start with the things that happen while you're drunk. We've all done stupid things that have created extra stress for ourselves. When you're hungover, you feel awful, making it harder to cope with the ups and downs of day-to-day life.

The more reliant you become on alcohol, the more stressed you feel about it. You're constantly wrestling with yourself about when you'll let yourself drink again, what you'll have and how much. And to top it all off, you've got the stress of knowing you have a drinking problem and all the emotions that brings with it!

Alcohol makes stress more likely to stick around because you're trying to mask the symptoms, rather than proactively deal with the root cause. Stress happens for a reason – it's often a sign that something is wrong and we need to pay attention.

#71
THE DRUNK VERSION OF YOU IS STILL YOU

Perhaps you're convinced that you're the life and soul of the party after your third gin and tonic, or that the drunk version of you is happier, friendlier and less anxious. The idea that we transform into different people when we're under the influence is a popular one. It turns out, though, that "drunk you" might not be as much of a thing as you think.

A study by the University of Missouri concluded that alcohol does not change our personality, it just creates a louder, more extroverted version of what is already there. While participants in the study reported feeling very affected by alcohol, observers didn't perceive such drastic changes. The point is, whether you think you're a mean drunk or a happy drunk, a funny boozer or just someone who becomes mellow and chilled out, the chances are this drunk version of you is pretty similar to the sober model.

#72
YOU DON'T NEED TO DRINK IN ORDER TO HAVE FUN

Alcohol companies often sponsor things that make us feel good, so we start to make the link between watching football and drinking beer, or laughing at a comedy show and drinking wine. You're being trained to think the two must go together when they absolutely don't!

I've always loved going to the theatre and seeing live music and comedy, but I find these activities so much better now I don't drink. When you're fully present and engaged (rather than thinking about your next drink or missing the show because you're queuing at the bar), you have so much more fun.

Just think about the parties you've been to where you had lots to drink, but no matter how drunk you were, you still didn't have a good time. Perhaps you were bored, got into a stupid argument or missed out on some of the fun because you were too zombified to notice. The reality is that drinking at a bad party just means you're drunk at a bad party.

#73
SOBER PEOPLE ARE NOT DULL

Stamp out any thoughts that you're a boring, sober loser – you aren't! Instead, examine your drinking over the past three months. Consider all the drinking occasions and the hangovers the next day. What opportunities have you missed out on as a result of your drinking? What have you not bothered to do because you felt rubbish? The chances are that alcohol is quietly making your life dull without you even realizing it.

When I look back on my drinking days, the thing that really stands out is how repetitive and boring they were. Drinking kept me stuck in a rut, doing the same thing over and over. It's no wonder I needed to consume a mind-altering drug in order to feel better about myself.

#74
LOOK TO THE CELEBRITIES

Hollywood might be associated with a champagne lifestyle, but there are lots of famous faces who are quietly teetotal. In an incredibly competitive industry, some of the most successful people on the planet have got to where they are because they don't waste their time, money, health and energy on alcohol.

A quick Internet search will bring up lots of articles about sober celebrities. Read through a few and see which stars resonate with you. Find out more about them or follow them on social media. Do they look like they're living terribly dull, miserable lives where they're never able to party, have fun or enjoy themselves? Go and see for yourself. This is all part of challenging the assumptions you've made about alcohol.

#75
BE AWARE OF YOUR CONFIRMATION BIAS

We all have a tendency to interpret events in a way that confirms our preconceptions. So, for example, if you decide that drinking wine is glamorous, you will subconsciously seek out information that supports this belief. And you'll conveniently forget – or not see – evidence that contradicts it.

My stop drinking course, Getting Unstuck, is six weeks long and, during that time, many of my students will experience their first night out sober. When they report back the next day, they often mention how shocked they were to spot other teetotallers or people who hardly drank anything.

When you're drinking, you look for other people who are boozing heavily, because it's reassuring. You become blind to the number of people who are quietly sober. And yet when you quit, these people are much more obvious! It's a bit like buying a new car – suddenly you spot cars just like yours everywhere. Of course, your car hasn't suddenly become really popular. You're simply noticing it more.

You will have some beliefs about booze which are false, but right now they *feel* true to you. Be aware of this and be open to changing your beliefs.

#76
PICTURE A CHILD IN YOUR SITUATION

Isn't it strange how we just expect children to cope with situations that we ourselves find difficult? We assume they'll settle in at a new school, make new friends and navigate all the other dramas that come with growing up in a scary world.

If a child was struggling with their homework or a relationship, we wouldn't crack open the wine for them, would we? The next time you're tempted to drink after a bad day, think about how you'd look after and comfort a child who was in the same situation. If you wouldn't give them a drug like alcohol, why are you giving it to yourself?

#77
LET YOUR EMOTIONS IN

The addiction expert Dr Gabor Maté says, "The attempt to escape from pain is what creates more pain." We live in a world that is obsessed with smothering emotions, particularly negative feelings. Whether we numb with alcohol or food, social media, gambling or shopping, we're trying to achieve the same effect: escape.

Know that whatever you're feeling right now is OK. It needs to be felt. Your mind and body are trying to tell you something. Perhaps something in your life does need to change, or you need to process certain feelings and experiences. This kind of work is tough and may take time, but it's worth it. This is how you create a life you genuinely feel good about; one that's so good, you don't need to numb your way through it.

#78
IT'S OK FOR SOBER FIRSTS TO BE TOUGH

The first time you do something is always the hardest. There's the first trip to the pub where you stick to soft drinks, the first date night without wine, the first sober work party. The first time is always the hardest because you're (a) nervous and (b) you're breaking an old association.

Know that this is all going to get so much easier. I bet there's something that's bothering you today, that in a few weeks' time you'll look back on and think, "I can't believe I was so worried about that!" Take comfort in the knowledge that how you feel is going to keep changing with time. This is one of the reasons you're taking a proper break from booze, so you can stick with it long enough to get to the good bit!

#79
BE A SOBER REBEL

I know that going against the crowd can feel tough. We all want to be accepted, right? But take it from someone who spent years trying to fit in and stay under the radar: breaking away from the norm sets you up for all kinds of good things.

When you really think about it, the fact that drinking is still "cool" is rather bizarre. There's nothing cool about being a sheep and following the crowd! Don't be embarrassed about being different or standing out. Be proud of it.

#80
FOCUS ON THE RIGHT THING

You're in control of your mindset and you can choose how you feel about alcohol-free living. You can tell yourself that it's dull, boring and hard. You can focus on what you believe you're missing out on. Or you can view alcohol-free living as a massive lifestyle upgrade instead.

Shift your attention to everything you're *gaining* during your break from booze. You're going to look better, feel happier, boost your energy, save money, beat anxiety *and* lose those horrible hangovers. Honestly, if you could buy a pill that did even half the things sobriety does, it would probably sell for thousands. Sobriety isn't about what you're missing out on – it's about what you're gaining.

MAKING
CHANGE
STICK

Sobriety is like wearing a new pair of boots: strange and uncomfortable at first, but after a while you can't imagine walking anywhere without them. I hope your break from booze has got off to a great start and you're beginning to feel the benefits of a hangover-free lifestyle. In this chapter, I want to talk about how to keep yourself motivated as the days turn into weeks. We'll also discuss what to do when you reach your sober goal, so you have a plan for moving forward.

#81
TRACK YOUR PROGRESS

There's something incredibly satisfying about being able to measure your progress with cold, hard facts and stats. Download a sobriety app onto your phone, so you can track how long you've been sober and how much money you've saved.

There are lots of different free apps out there, but I like the Sober Time app because it also delivers daily motivational quotes. Another good app is I'm Done Drinking, which tells you how many drinks you've not had and how many calories you've saved.

If you wear a fitness tracker, keep an eye on your daily step count, resting heart rate and the quality of your sleep each night. An unexpected side effect of sobriety is that you tend to sleep better, exercise more and feel healthier in general. If you're a numbers geek like me, and you've been wearing your fitness tracker for a while, it can be very interesting to observe the impact sobriety has on your overall health.

#82
CELEBRATE THE UNEXPECTED

In early sobriety, you're bound to notice a few surprising benefits that you hadn't anticipated. Perhaps you no longer have a bulging recycling bin, full of empties. Maybe you have more patience with your kids and fewer arguments with your partner. Perhaps your skin is better because the sober you makes time for a proper skincare routine before bed. Celebrate these smaller, unexpected side effects of sobriety, because they all add up!

#83
KEEP AN "I DID IT" LIST

Whenever you successfully tackle something tricky without drinking, write it down. It doesn't matter what it is – anything that feels like a win, big or small, should go on your list! There are two reasons why it's really important to do this. First, the things that feel like challenges today soon won't be. You'll quickly move your attention on to something else. You'll forget that once upon a time, not drinking on a Friday night felt like a really big deal.

The second reason is that when you do go through a tough time, it's useful to look back on your list and remind yourself of what you've already been through. This list is proof that you can do hard things and you're capable of more than you think.

#84
CREATE A SOBRIETY PHOTO ALBUM

Take pictures of anything that reminds you of a good sober moment. It might be a snap of the flowers you bought yourself with the money you saved on booze. It could be a picture of the homework you patiently helped your kids finish because you were fully present and sober. Or perhaps you did a fun activity together that wouldn't have happened if you'd been hungover.

Pictures are a great way to record your sober highlights. Keep the photos in an album on your phone, so you can revisit them whenever you need a pick-me-up or a reminder of exactly why you're doing this.

Note: You can also flip this around and create a "negative" photo album if you find that more powerful. Some people like visual reminders of what happens when they drink and what they're leaving behind.

#85
TAKE SELFIES!

Did you remember to take a picture of yourself at the beginning of your break from booze? I hope so! Now's the time to take another one. You may not notice a difference on a day-to-day basis, but I think you'll be surprised by the changes you observe when you're looking at these pictures side by side.

Your eyes might be a little whiter and brighter. Perhaps you look less tired because you've been sleeping better. Without alcohol, your skin might look healthier and less puffy. Keep taking these photos every few weeks so you can observe further changes over time.

#86
TAME YOUR SOCIAL MEDIA

It's not helpful to see tons of posts about drinking or memes about wine o'clock every time you log on to Facebook or Instagram. We spend so much time online these days, it's important that our news feeds don't make us feel drained or left out.

Unfollow or mute people who constantly post about alcohol – they won't even know you've done it. Experiment with moving social media apps away from the front page of your phone and turning notifications off.

You could also consider creating a separate account that's completely sobriety related. Make it a safe little bubble full of inspiring quotes and things that motivate you. Come and follow me – I'm @thesoberschool on Instagram, Facebook and Twitter.

#87

"IT WOULD NEVER HAVE HAPPENED TO ME IF I'D BEEN DRINKING."

What experiences have you had during your break that simply wouldn't have happened without sobriety? Write a list. I asked some of my Getting Unstuck students to answer this question and here's what they said:

> " I trusted myself to have my one-year-old granddaughter stay overnight. This is something I've really enjoyed. "
>
> – *Dianne*

> " I've seen the look of pride in my daughter's eyes every time she sees me return from an event totally alcohol free. "
>
> – *Jackie*

> " I graduated my masters program with a 4.0! "
>
> – *Elizabeth*

" I wake up each morning well rested, rock the early morning barre class and I'm at the office by 8 a.m. ready to take on the day. "

— *Bee*

" I published my first book! I had been trying to finish this for eight years. Being alcohol free unleashed my creative energy. "

— *Cheryl*

" I bought a horse with the money I saved! Owning a horse has always been one of the things on my to do list ... and now I'm not drinking, I have the time to do it. "

— *Jane*

#88
THE BIG DECISION – WHAT WILL YOU DO NEXT?

Once you hit your goal and reach the end of your break from booze, you have a big decision to make: what will your next move be? Do you want to go back to drinking, or set another short-term goal and extend your break? It's completely up to you.

To help you with your decision, I recommend you review the list you wrote outlining the reasons why you wanted to take this break in the first place. Remind yourself of the reality of your drinking and how alcohol affects you. Journal about how you're feeling now and make a list of everything that makes you feel proud. Look at your selfies, your "I did it" list and your sobriety tracker app for inspiration.

If you wish to continue with alcohol-free living, I suggest setting another achievable, short-term goal. You don't need to be ready to stop drinking forever. (That can be a very intimidating and overwhelming prospect!) Setting smaller, doable goals will keep you moving forward until you reach a point where you no longer need to set them. For me, this happened around the one-year mark – that's when I knew that I wanted to stay alcohol free for good.

#89
THERE ARE ONLY TWO CHOICES

Time for some tough love here. As you contemplate what to do next, it's important to understand that you're only choosing between two options. You can continue with alcohol-free living or go back to drinking in exactly the same way as you were before. There is no magic middle path of moderation. If moderation worked for you, you wouldn't be reading this book.

Here's what will happen if you try moderation after your break. To start with, things will probably feel fine. Your tolerance to the drug will be low, so you'll feel the effects quickly and it might feel easy to stop after one or two. You'll probably think, "Ah ha! Kate Bee got it wrong. Look at me. I am in control."

But after one drinking episode, you'll want to do it again. You'll have fed the booze monster – the part of you that believes you can't be happy without this drug in your life. Eventually you'll drink again, your tolerance will rise and soon you'll be back to where you started.

Over the years I've worked with thousands of people and I do not know of a single person who has morphed into a carefree, happy and satisfied moderate drinker. Moderation is such hard work – it drains your energy. In the long term, it can be soul-destroying. You have been warned!

#90
DON'T BE AFRAID TO MAKE OTHER CHANGES

The clarity that comes with sobriety can shine a light on other aspects of your life which aren't working as well as they could be. If you decide to extend your break from booze, you have the perfect opportunity to make a few other changes. This goes back to something I mentioned earlier. In sobriety, we're trying to create a life that truly works, that feels good – so good you don't need to take a mind-numbing drug in order to cope with it.

When I quit, one of the things I realized I needed to change was my job. It suddenly became obvious that I wasn't in the right career, and it wasn't something I was willing to keep ignoring or putting up with. In fact, I could see that work had created a lot of stress for me and exacerbated my drinking. Finding a new job and carving out a new career wasn't something that happened quickly, but it's a project I began tackling early in my sobriety.

#91
LOOK AT WHO YOU'RE SURROUNDING YOURSELF WITH

The motivational speaker Jim Rohn famously said, "We are the average of the five people we spend the most time with." We are greatly influenced by those closest to us, whether we like it or not. It affects our way of thinking, our self-esteem and our decisions. So, who are the five people you hang out with the most?

Are they positive influences in your life or are they holding you back? Are they your true friends, or just drinking buddies? Do they support your sobriety, or are they tearing it down? We only get one life, so make sure you're spending quality time with people who genuinely care about you.

#92
DON'T LET LONELINESS BE A TRIGGER

I often drank because I was lonely, and I've noticed this issue comes up with my clients too. Many of us move around for work, and making friends as an adult can be tough. Technology might make us feel as if we're "connected" to those around us, but a few likes and shares on social media isn't true friendship.

If you suspect you might have been drinking because you're bored or lonely, I highly recommend making the effort to take up a new hobby and get out and meet new people. Commit to doing one thing a week and see how you go. You could take an evening class, join a running club or learn a new hobby. Meetup.com is a great website for finding activities in your area.

#93
READ SOME SELF-HELP BOOKS

When you've been drinking to escape certain feelings, or even yourself, it's a sign that something isn't quite right. The clear-headedness sobriety brings is a great time to explore what those issues are.

Let's face it – it's hard to be an adult in today's world without having some hang-ups about ourselves. When we're not smothering our feelings with a mind-numbing substance, we give ourselves a chance to work through these issues instead. If you're not sure where to start, here are three books I recommend:

- *You Are a Badass*, Jen Sincero

- *Daring Greatly*, Brené Brown

- *I Heart Me*, David Hamilton

#94

DON'T STRESS ABOUT SUGAR CRAVINGS

Alcoholic drinks can contain a lot of sugar, so when you cut booze out of your diet, your body may crave the sweet stuff. Sugar, like alcohol, can temporarily raise serotonin and dopamine levels in the brain (your feel-good brain chemicals).

Do not worry about sugar cravings or put yourself on a punishing diet. The most important thing is that you're not drinking – that's all that matters in early sobriety. Time and patience will heal your sugar cravings, as you adjust to alcohol-free living and become more comfortable in your sober shoes. (This is yet another reason for taking a proper break from booze!)

Focus on eating nourishing, regular meals and filling your plate with protein, healthy fats and leafy greens. Plan a healthy snack for late afternoon. Get plenty of sleep and some gentle exercise. And that's it. If you want to indulge your sweet tooth between meals, go for it. This too shall pass.

#95
WHAT TO DO IF YOU SLIP UP

We like to think success is a smooth path from A to B, but it rarely is. If you drink during your break from booze, the most important thing is to get straight back up again and keep going. Don't beat yourself up or decide that this is impossible.

Instead, reflect on why you drank and what benefit you thought the drug would give you. What sober tools could you have used instead? If you were able to live the same day over again, what would you do differently? Try to learn from what happened, so you can avoid making the same mistake again.

Success is not about doing something perfectly, without failure. It's about having the courage to do it in the first place. If we only ever did things that we were sure we wouldn't fail at, we wouldn't get very far, would we? Try and see a slip for what it really is: a lesson learned, a bump in the road. It's a chance to review what's working and what's not – and then move on.

#96
START A GRATITUDE DIARY

Gratitude might sound cheesy, but tests at the University of California found that people who kept a gratitude journal for just three weeks measured 25% higher on life satisfaction. They exercised more, drank less alcohol and their families and friends noticed they were nicer to be around.

When you're feeling negative – and your focus is on everything you don't have, or can't have – you're going to feel less motivated. You're far more likely to hit wine o'clock and think, "What's the point?" Training your brain to be more positive will help you stay motivated.

Today I am grateful for…

1. ....
   ....
   ....
   ....
   ....
   ....
   ....
   ....
   ....

2. ....
   ....
   ....
   ....
   ....
   ....
   ....
   ....
   ....

3. ....
   ....
   ....
   ....
   ....
   ....
   ....
   ....
   ....

#97
CREATE NEW TRADITIONS

We all have habits and patterns that show up in different ways throughout our lives. Perhaps you always have wine and pizza on a Friday night to mark the end of the working week. If the thought of not having wine makes you feel deprived, now's the time to create a brand new tradition instead. Don't put up with feeling like you're missing out!

Perhaps Friday nights could become movie night – you could head out to the cinema or watch a movie at home. Set up a mocktail bar that the whole family can enjoy. Or go out and do an activity together. Friday nights could become quality family time that you commit to, no matter what. Trust your gut here – go with what feels good.

#98
FLASH THE CASH

Alcohol-free living should be a massive lifestyle upgrade, so make sure your wallet has got the message! By not drinking, you're saving quite a bit of money and you shouldn't be afraid to spend it on yourself.

Now is a great time to think about the things you don't enjoy doing and would love to hire out. A few bottles of wine a week would cover the cost of a cleaner or someone to tackle the ironing. Or you could put the money toward a meal delivery service, personal training sessions or a hobby you've always wanted to try.

#99
HAVE NO REGRETS

If you're ever feeling unsure about what to do next, or you're struggling to stay motivated, I hope you find comfort in this thought: No one ever regrets waking up hangover free. Seriously. No one ever rolls over and thinks, "I really wish I'd drunk loads last night!"

When you're alcohol free, you have far fewer regrets in general. You don't spend time regretting the opportunities you missed when you were too hungover to care; you don't beat yourself up about what you said the night before, how much you had to drink, or the promises to yourself that you broke. Don't ever forget how good it feels to be free of that worry and anxiety.

#100
BE PROUD

Congratulations for taking a break from booze and having the courage to step outside your comfort zone! You should feel hugely proud of yourself for taking action and trying something different.

Please remember this: sobriety is nothing to be embarrassed about or ashamed of. It's not something you need to hide or keep secret. I hope this lifestyle makes you feel proud and happy – it's a brilliant gift to give yourself and you deserve to feel great about it.

Ultimately, alcohol-free living is about freedom. Without booze holding you back, you're free to do the things you truly want to do, and be the best version of yourself. You're free from the endless obsession with alcohol, and free to be fully present in your one and only life.

So here's to freedom – and to many more amazing, alcohol-free days ahead.

INDEX

RESOURCES

Further reading:
<u>Self-help books</u>
You Are a Badass, Jen Sincero
Daring Greatly, Brené Brown
I Heart Me, David Hamilton

<u>Books about sobriety</u>
Kick The Drink... Easily!, Jason Vale
The Unexpected Joy of Being Sober, Catherine Gray
The Sober Diaries, Clare Pooley

Podcasts:
The Bubble Hour
Real women sharing real stories of recovery from addiction.

Take a Break From Drinking
Hosted by life coach Rachel Hart.

The Alcohol-Free Life Podcast
Inspiring interviews with BBC Radio 2 presenter Janey Lee Grace.

Alcohol-free drinks:
Drydrinker.com
A great website with an inspiring selection of alcohol-free drinks.

Clubsodaguide.com
Great for finding places that serve low and no alcohol drinks.

Dry, Clare Liardet
Interested in mocktails but not sure where to start? This book is
    packed with inspiration.

Apps:
Sober Time
Tracks your sobriety and shares a daily motivational quote.

I'm Done Drinking
Tracks your days, number of drinks not consumed and the number of
    calories saved!

Inspiring Instagram accounts:
@thesoberschool
Of course I would recommend myself!

@tellbetterstoriesmedia
Great at highlighting silly marketing messages about alcohol.

@mrs_d_alcoholfree
I love Lotta Dann's posts – she's the author of *Mrs D Is Going
    Without*.